Latifa MTIBAA
Ameni HAGGARI
Boutheina JEMLI

Retrospective study of vulvovaginal candidiasis

Latifa MTIBAA
Ameni HAGGARI
Boutheina JEMLI

Retrospective study of vulvovaginal candidiasis

ScienciaScripts

Imprint

Cover image: www.ingimage.com

This book is a translation from the original published under ISBN 978-620-3-41239-0.

Publisher:
Sciencia Scripts
is a trademark of
International Book Market Service Ltd., member of OmniScriptum Publishing Group
17 Meldrum Street, Beau Bassin 71504, Mauritius
Printed at: see last page
ISBN: 978-620-3-38784-1

Retrospective study of vulvovaginal candidiasis

Author: Dr MTIBAA Latifa

Summary

List of Abbreviations

CVV: Vulvo-Vaginal Candidiasis

HMPIT: Main Military Training Hospital of Tunis

Fig : Figure

IUD: Intrauterine Device

ALS: Agglutinin-Like

Sequences **Hwp1:** Hyphal

Wall Protein

EPM: Extracellular Polysaccharide Matrix

PCB: Potato Core-Bile

RAT: Riz-Agar-Tween

AT: Agar-Tween

S: Sabouraud

SC: Sabouraud chloramphenicol

SCA: Sabouraud chloramphenicol Actidione

SF: Sun Flower

MIC: minimal inhibitory concentration

T: Trimester of pregnancy

List of Figures

List of Tables

Abstract

Introduction

Vulvo-vaginal candidiasis (CVV) is a symptomatic genital mycosis caused by yeasts of the *Candida* genus. It affects approximately 75% of women with genital activity. The aim of our study was to determine the prevalence of CVV and to describe its epidemiological and mycological profile.

Materials and methods

This is a retrospective study that included 1058 vaginal swabs collected during three months between October and December 2018 in the laboratory of Parasitology-Mycology of the main military hospital of instruction in Tunis. For each sample, a direct examination with systematic culture on Sabouraud medium (S), S-chloramphenicol (SC), and SC-actidione medium (SCA) was performed. The identification of the pathogen is made by the chlamydosporulation test, API 20Cand vitek2 YST ID The antifungigram is performed using the vitek2 AST ID and the E-test for 2 samples at the request of the clinician.

Results

Out of a total of 1058 samples received, 273 were culture positive, for an overall prevalence of 25.8%. The mean age of the patients is 32 years (± 6.91) with extremes of 20 to 64 years. In 67.3% of the cases the women were pregnant, particularly during the first trimester (46.3%). Leucorrhoea was the most frequent symptom (57.6%) followed by vulvar pruritus (40.2%), and urinary burning (16.8%). The sensitivity of direct examination was 68.5%. The species isolated were *Candida albicans* (66%), *C. glabrata* (26.7%), *C. krusei* (3.1%), *C. Tropicalis* (2.1%). *C.parapsilosis* (1.7%) and *C.dubliniensis* (0.4%). One *Candida albicans strain* and one *Candida glabrata* strain were sensitive to voriconazole, flucytosine, caspofungin, micafungin and amphotericin B. For fluconazole, *C.albicans* was sensitive but *C.glabrata* was intermediate.

Conclusion

Our study shows that VSC is a frequent reason for women to consult a doctor. Its diagnosis results from the comparison of the mycological examination with anamnestic and clinical data. Mycological diagnosis is a key element in the management of this infection.

Abstract

Introduction

Vulvovaginal candidiasis (VVC) is a symptomatic genital mycosis caused by yeasts genus *Candida*. It affects about 75% of women in genital activity. The purpose of our study was to determine the prevalence of VVC and describe their epidemiological and mycological profile.

Methods

This retrospective study included 1058 vaginal samples collected during three months between October and December 2018 in the laboratory of Parasitology-Mycology of military hospital of Tunis. For each sample, a direct examination with culture on Sabouraud (S) medium, S-chloramphenicol (SC), and SC-actidione medium (SCA) were performed. The identification of the pathogen is made the chlamydosporulation test, API 20C and vitek2 YST ID . Susceptibility to antifungals is tested using vitek 2 AST ID card and E-test for 2 samples at the request of the clinician.

Results

Among total of 1058 samples received, 273 presented a positive culture, giving an overall prevalence of 25.8%. The average age of patients is 32 (± 6,91) years with extremes of 20 to 64 years. In 67.3% of cases women were pregnant and particularly in the first trimester (46.3%). Leucorrhea was the most common symptom (57.6%) followed by vulvo-vaginal pruritus (40.2%) and urinary burning (16.8%). The sensitivity of direct examination was 68.5%. The isolated species were *Candida albicans* (66%), *C. glabrata* (26.7%), *C. krusei* (3.1%), *C. Tropicalis* (2.1%). *C.parapsilosis* (1.7%) and *C.dubliniensis* (0.4%). One isolate of *Candida albicans* and one of *Candida glabrata* were susceptible to voriconazole, flucytosine, caspofungin, micafungin and amphotericin B. For fluconazole, *C.albicans* was sucsceptible but *C. glabrata* was intermediate.

Conclusion

Our study shows that VVC is a frequent reason for women's consultation. His diagnosis results from confrontation of anamnestic, clinical and mycological data. Mycological examination is key element in management of this infection.

General Introduction

Introduction

Infectious vulvo-vaginitis is a common condition that manifests itself as vulvar and/or vaginal irritation due to microorganisms **(Hedayati et *al* . , 2015)** **(Kechia et *al* . , 2015)**. Among the latter are fungi that can go from commensalism to pathogenicity, such as *Candida* yeasts **(Papon et *al*.,2013)**. In fact, this microorganism is part of the mucosal flora of most healthy women that proliferate and colonize the vulvo-vaginal system **(Rodriguez- Cerdeira et *al*.,2018)**.

Candida vaginitis or vulvovaginal candidiasis (CVV) is the second most common cause of infectious vaginitis after bacterial vaginosis **(Mtibaa et *al*.,2017)**. **CVV** is considered a fungal opportunistic infection linked to local dysfunction of cellular immunity **(El Euch et *al*.,2014)**. It is not a sexually transmitted disease **(Ogouyèmi-Hounto et *al*.,2014)**. It affects women during the reproductive period as well as diabetic and immunodeficient patients. Vaginitis is generally associated with considerable morbidity, healthcare costs, distress, pain and sexual dysfunction **(Seifi et al.,2015)** and can even lead to infertility **(Hedayati et *al*.,2015)**. Thus, it significantly reduces the quality of life of young women, with a strong negative impact on their work and social life **(Hedayati et *al*.,2015)**. The objective of our study is to determine the prevalence of CVV in a Tunisian population, to describe their clinical (leucorrhoea, vulvar pruritus and urinary tract burn) and mycological aspects, and to evaluate the sensitivity of certain *Candida* species to antifungal agents.

Bibliographic synthesis

1. Vaginal flora

1.1. Anatomy and Physiology of the Female Genitalia

The genital system includes two types of organs: the internal genitals (vagina, uterus, fallopian tubes and ovaries) and the external organs or vulva **(Bougahanmi, 2015).**

This anatomy is illustrated in **Figure 1.**

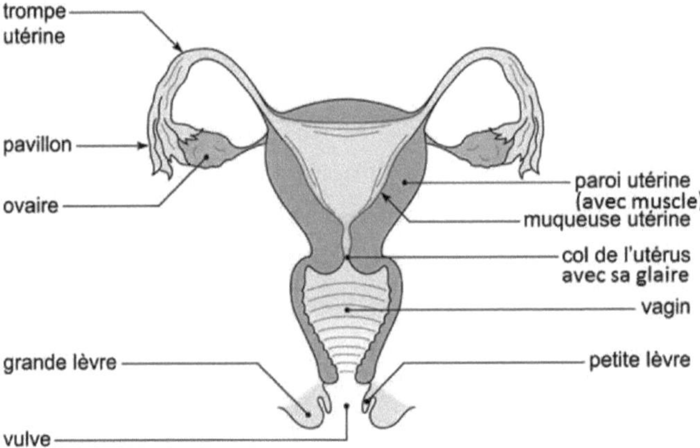

Figure 1. The female genitalia in frontal section **(Bougahanmi, 2015).**

The female genital tract is made up of two distinct sectors separated by the cervix from a microbiological point of view. The first is located at the top and is sterile due to the action of cervical mucus, which presents an impassable barrier for microorganisms **(Bougahanmi, 2015).**

While the vulva, vagina and in some cases the ectocervix constitute the female genital mucosa. These anatomical sites are particularly susceptible to infection **(D Parent, 2017).**

1.2. Vaginal pH

The pH of the vagina of healthy women is acidic, ranging from 3.8 to 4.5 measured at the lateral and anterior cul-de-sacs of the vagina. This acidity provides protection against vaginal infections **(Godha et *al.,* 2017).**

Many factors contribute to the successive variation of vaginal pH including hormones, composition of the vaginal microbiota **(Godha et *al.,* 2017).** This acidic environment is provided by lactobacilli by producing lactic acid **(Greenbaum et *al.*, 2018).**

The shift to a higher alkaline pH reduces the viability of healthy endogenous vaginal microbiota, while encouraging the growth of pathogenic Gram-negative fecal flora and other bacterial species **(Godha et *al.*, 2017).**

1.3. Composition of the normal microbial flora

The normal vaginal flora often includes hemolytic streptococci, anaerobic streptococci *(Pepto Streptococci),* bacteroid species, *Clostridia, Gardnerella spp, Ureaplasma urealyticum* and sometimes *Listeria* or *Mobiluncus* species **(Masand et *al.,* 2015).** Most of them are not harmful **(Greenbaum et *al.*, 2018).**

In addition, the vaginal microbiota of a normal woman of childbearing age is characterized by the dominance of gram-positive beneficial bacteria such as *Lactobacillus*:
L. crispatus, L. gasseri, L. iners and L. jensenii which are essential producers of lactic acid by glycogen fermentation **(Tachedjian et *al.*, 2017).**

1.4. Variability of the vaginal flora

The vaginal microbial ecosystem can be influenced by many physiological factors such as the menstrual cycle, pregnancy, menopause and other hormonal changes **(Greenbaum et *al.,* 2018).**

- **At puberty:** Because of the rise in estrogen levels leading to a thickening of the vaginal mucosa responsible for the increase in glycogen content **(Ogouyèmi-Hounto et *al.,* 2014)**, this period is characterized by an abundance of *lactobacilli* **(Miller et *al.*, 2016).**
- During the menstrual **cycle:** The stability of the microbial community decreases

during menstruation and correlates with low estrogen levels. Indeed the abundance of *Gardnerella vaginalis* increases during menstruation with a concomitant decrease in *Lactobacillus* species, excluding *Lactobacillus iners*. This can be explained by the lysis of vaginal blood during menstruation and increased iron levels, which support the accelerated growth of *G. vaginalis* and *L. iners* **(Greenbaum et *al.*, 2018).**

- During **pregnancy:** This period is characterized by high *lactobacillus* levels **(Greenbaum et *al.*, 2018)** since the level of secreted hormones (progesterone and estrogen) increases considerably **(Amouri et *al.*, 2010).**
- During the **menopause:** the vaginal flora is poor in *lactobacilli* but rich in anaerobes (*Bacteroides*, *Mobiluncus*) and the same for *G. vaginalis* because of a decrease in estrogen secretion **(Greenbaum et *al.*, 2018).**

2. Vulvovaginal candidiasis

Vulvo-vaginal candidiasis is an infectious vaginitis caused by yeasts of the *Candida* genus **(Kechia et *al.*, 2015).**

2.1. Physiopathology

Candida spp is an opportunistic yeast that is part of the vaginal flora in 10-20% of healthy women of childbearing age **(Rodríguez-Cerdeira et *al.*, 2018).** Indeed, it can change from commensal to pathogenic state as a result of a disturbance in the balance between the host immune system in the vaginal mucosa and the virulence mechanisms of this fungus. Thus, in candidiasis infection, three stages must be distinguished **(De Chauvin, 2009)**:

- **Commensalism or saprophytism:** *Candida* is present as blastospores in small quantities and in balance with the local flora of other microorganisms.
- **Colonization:** At this stage, *Candida* is present in larger quantities but retains its blastospore form without pseudo-filaments (**Fig.2**).

This results in an abnormal local situation such as vaginal dryness.

- **Pathogenicity:** Infection (or genital candidiasis): yeast multiplication and filamentation (**Fig.2) causing** inflammatory lesions of the vaginal mucosa.

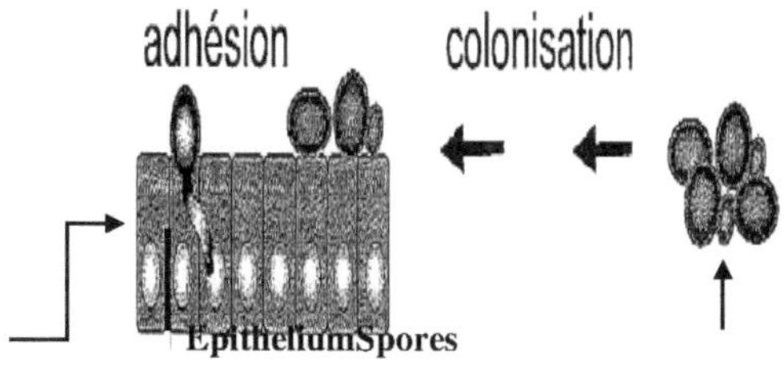

Figure 2. Pathophysiopathology of mucocutaneous candidiasis **(Eggimann and Pittet ,2002)**

2.2. Favouring factors

2.2.1. Intrinsic factors

- **Hormonal impregnation**

VVC is hormone-dependent **(Amouri et *al.* , 2010). Indeed,** estrogens have a multifunctional and permissive role for CVV, especially during pregnancy characterized by hormonal imbalance **(Cassone, 2014).** This modification leads to a decrease in vaginal pH, which favours the implantation of *Candida* yeasts. In fact, the increase in estrogen levels during this period provides an excellent source of carbon for *Candida* via the production of glycogen, ensuring their multiplication and adhesion to epithelial cells **(Amouri et *al.,* 2010) (Ogouyèmi-Hounto et *al.,* 2014).**

- **Diabetes**

Uncontrolled diabetes predisposes to VSC **(Amouri et *al.,* 2010).** The presence of glucose in the vaginal secretions of diabetic patients constitutes a nutritive source for yeast and promotes its adherence, growth and expression of virulence factors. Indeed, hyperglycemia leads to monocyte and phagocytosis insufficiency and limits the ability of neutrophils to eliminate the pathogen **(Amouri et *al.,* 2010) (Van Schalkwyk et *al.*, 2015).**

- **Immune factors**

An immune deficiency due to situations such as HIV infection promotes the incidence of VVC. Indeed, HIV-positive women, as well as women with other forms of immunosuppression, are more frequently affected by CVV but are not the most severe **(Amouri et *al.*, 2010).**

- **Local factors**

Maceration, humidity and containment are factors that promote yeast growth and proliferation. As a result, the wearing of too tight and synthetic clothing favours *Candida* infection (**Amouri et *al.*, 2010).** In addition, intimate hygiene, particularly anal hygiene from the anus to the vagina, promotes the development of CVV. According to studies by **Holanda et al (2007),** patients colonized by *Candida albicans* in the anus are five times more likely to develop CVV.

2.2.2. Extrinsic (iatrogenic) factors

- **Antibiotic therapy** seems to be associated with the destruction of the bacterial microbiota, particularly *lactobacilli, which* favours the appearance of CVV **(Holanda et *al.*, 2007).**
- **Immunosuppressive therapeutics** such as corticotherapy, radiotherapy and chemotherapy play a major role in the development of vulvovaginal infections **(Amouri et *al.*, 2010).**
- The use of high-dose **oral contraceptives** or **hormone replacement therapy** leads to an increase in glycogen, which is the nutritional substrate of yeast, since these are hyperestrogenic situations, hence the stimulation of vaginal mucosal infection **(Holanda et *al.*, 2007).**
- **Mechanical contraceptives** (intrauterine device (IUD), vaginal ring) contribute to the pathogenesis of VVC. Recent studies show that *C. albicans* has a high capacity to adhere and produce biofilm on the surface of the IUD, allowing it to evade host immunity and reduce their sensitivity to antifungal agents **(Amouri et *al.*, 2010).**

2.3. Species involved in VVC

2.3.1. General

Mushrooms (international name: Fungi) are single or multi-cellular eukaryotic organisms, devoid of chlorophyll, which clearly distinguishes it from the plant kingdom. However, they constitute a separate kingdom between the animal and plant worlds **(Develoux and Brittany, 2005).**

Yeasts are unicellular, yeast-like microscopic fungi, classified in two major phyla of fungi: ascomycetes and basidomycetes **(Defosse et *al.* , 2018).** They are mainly represented by *Candida* **(Develoux and Bretagne, 2005).**

2.3.2. Taxonomy

The *Candida* genus groups together yeasts whose majority of the characteristics are found in ascomycetes. This classification is based on phenotypic characters and on the comparison of nucleotide sequences **(Bougahanmi, 2015) (Defosse et *al.,* 2016).**

Kingdom : Mushroom

Phylum: Ascomycota

Class: Hemiacomyces

Order: Saccaromycetales (budding yeasts)

Family: Candidaceae

Genre: *Candida*

Species : *Candida albicans, glabrata, tropicalis, parapsilosis...*

2.3.3. Morphology

This genus gathers non-pigmented yeasts not capped giving creamy white colonies in culture. *Candida* cells have a rounded or oval shape and are heterotrophic (no photosynthesis). Their wall is composed of chitin and glycogen. Concerning the vegetative apparatus, it can take various forms: oval blastospores originating from multilateral budding, pseudo filament, filament, originating from parent yeasts (**Table 1**) **(Develoux & Bretagne, 2005).**

2.3.4. Antigenic structure

The wall of these yeasts consists of a more internal layer formed by a very dense network of polysaccharides (80%-90%) including chitin, β-1.3 glucans associated with β-1.6 glucans and proteins (mannoproteins) mainly on the external layer (**Fig. 3**) **(Rodríguez-Cerdeira et *al.,* 2018).** The richness of *Candida* in glycans (especially polysaccharides or polysaccharide antigens) gives species specificity. This specificity allows the initiation of the anti-Candida response by involving monoclonal and polyclonal antibodies **(Poulain, 2013).**

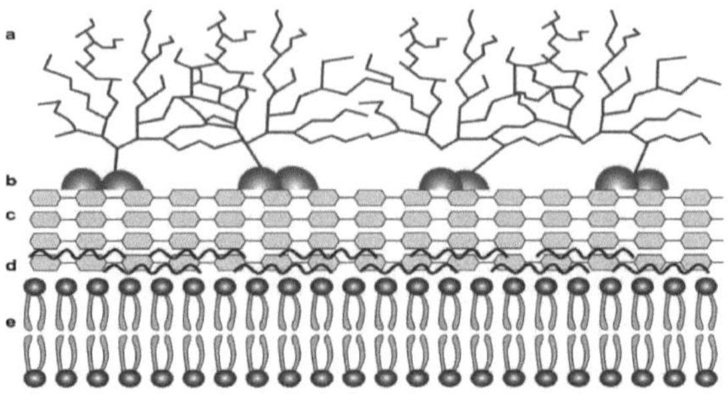

Figure 3: Diagram illustrating *Candida* cell walls **(Rodríguez-Cerdeira et *al.*,2018). a** fibril layer, **b** mannoproteins, **c** β glucans, **d** β glucans-chitin, **e** cytoplasmic membrane.

2.3.5. Ecological niche

Candida are endogenous or exogenous commensal microorganisms that are the most widely expressed in human pathology, counting 200 species **(Sharma et *al.*, 2019).** During their adaptation to commensalism, some species have specialized for certain anatomical sites. There are two forms of infection caused by *Candida*: superficial (cutaneous, unguous, oral, auricular, genitourinary) and disseminated or septicaemic (deep candidiasis) **(Develoux and Bretagne, 2005).** The specific anatomical sites for certain species, their morphology and the infection caused are presented in **Table 1.**

Table 1. Main *Candida* species involved in human pathology and their morphologies **(Develoux and Bretagne, 2005) (Sharma et *al.,* 2019).**

Species	Morphology	Saprophytic state	Event Clinic
C.albicans	Yeast, pseudohyphe, Hyphe	Digestive tract and genital system	Cutaneous mucosal candidiasis Digestive and urinary candidiasis Candidaemia, systemic candidiasis
C.glabrata	Yeast	Digestive tract and genitourinar y tract	Vaginitis, urinary candidiasis Candidaemia, candidiasis, systemic candidiasis
C.parapsilosis	Yeast, pseudohyph,	Skin	Applicants
C. tropicalis	Yeast, pseudohyphe, Hyphe	Commensal of the nature (soil, plants, water)	Vaginitis, Candidaemia, systemic candidiasis
C . kefyr	Yeast, pseudohyph,	Dairy products	Systemic candidiasis
C. krusei	Yeast, pseudohyph,	Dairy products and beer	Vaginitis, Candidaemia
C.dubliniensis	Yeast, Pseudohypha, Hyphe	Isolated in people with AIDS (oral cavity, lung, vagina, blood and excrement)	Oral candidiasis , Candidaemia

2.3.6. Virulence factors

Yeasts of the *Candida* genus have factors contributing to their good adaptation as a pathogen for humans **(Sharma et *al.,* 2019).** *Candida albicans* is considered the most virulent because of its multiple virulence factors **(Tsui et *al.,* 2016).**

2.3.6.1. Surface adhesives

The infectious process initially involves the adhesion of yeast to receptors in host tissues, which is promoted by the expression of a family of adhesins:

agglutinin-like sequences (ALS) **(Tsui et al., 2016)** associated with hyphae **(Defosse et *al.,* 2018).** This family is composed of eight proteins of which ALS3 is the most important. Similarly, there is another major adhesin of the hyphae wall (Hwp1) **(Tsui et *al.*, 2016).**

2.3.6.2. Biofilm

Biofilm occurs when a microorganism encounters an abiotic surface or host tissue **(Tsui et *al.,* 2016)** in a series of steps (**Fig.4**).

- ➤ **Adhesion A**: Adhesion of the yeasts forming a basal layer that implants the biofilm.
- ➤ Initiation **B**: Yeast proliferation in filamentous form.
- ➤ Maturation **C**: production of an extracellular polysaccharide matrix (EPM).
- ➤ Dispersion **D**: the yeasts are released from the biofilm, allowing the colonization of other surfaces.

This biofilm enables yeast resistance to antifungal treatments by inhibiting their diffusion **(Tsui et *al.,* 2016).**

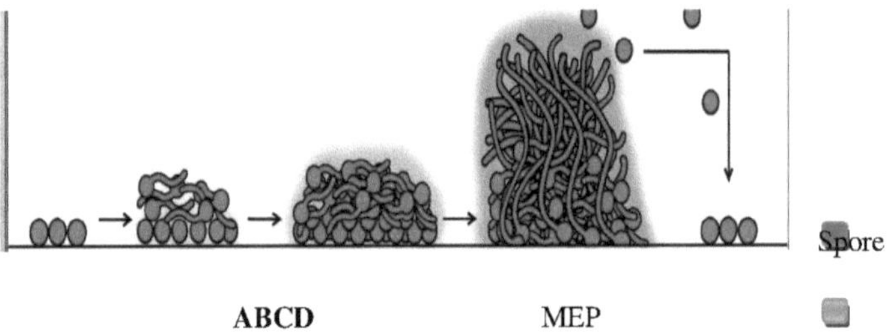

Figure 4. Development of Candida albicans biofilm **(Tsui et *al.,* 2016).**

2.3.6.3. Phenotypic switching (Dimorphic switch)

It is the ability to transform from the yeast form into a **mycelial** filament **(Palkova and Vachova, 2016),** in response to different environmental conditions such as temperature, pH level, CO_2 **(Tsui et *al.,* 2016),** hormonal imbalance **(Amouri et *al.,* 2010).** These two different forms are illustrated in **Figure 5.**

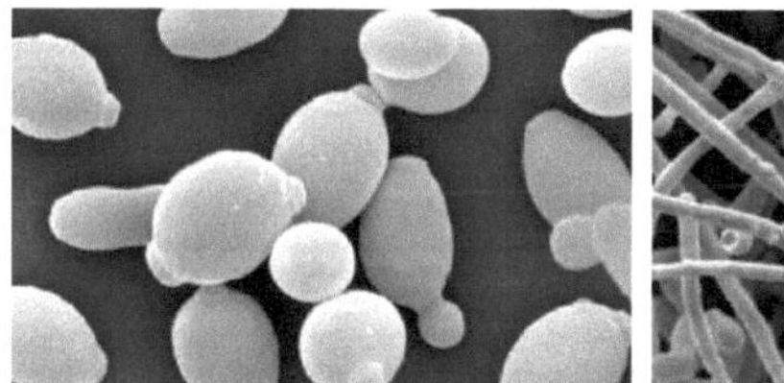 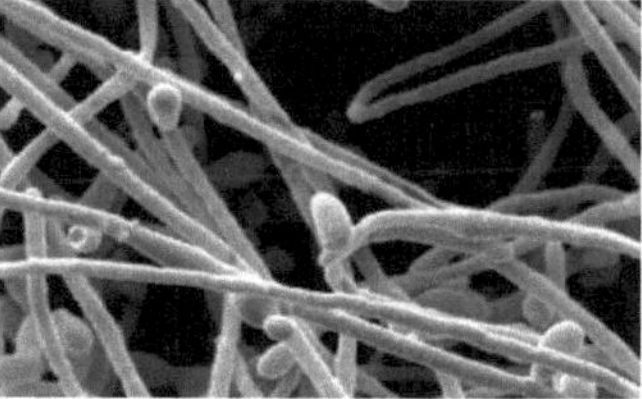

Figure 5: Baying electron micrograph of yeast cells (left) and hyphae (right) of *Candida albicans* **(Cassone, 2014).**

3. Mycological diagnosis of CVV

It consists of 4 steps: sampling, direct examination, culture and finally identification of the species by various tests based on morphological, immunological, biochemical and molecular criteria **(Pihet and Marot, 2013).**

3.1. Sampling

Ideally, two swabs are taken from the affected area, one for direct examination and one for mycological culture. However, if a single swab is used, it is recommended that it be suspended in a small amount of sterile distilled water or saline to perform both direct examination and culture **(Anofel et *al.,* 2017).**

3.2. Direct examination

ED is performed either directly in a fresh state by adding an uncolored liquid (distilled water or saline), or by using a dye that improves the visualization of blastoconidia: 2% lugol, toluidine blue, lactophenol blue, chlorazole black or congo red (MycetColor®, sr2b) **(Pihet and Marot, 2013).**

3.3. Culture

Sabouraud medium is the basic medium for the isolation and culture of fungi responsible for human mycosis. It is often enriched with simple carbohydrates (glucose, maltose, dextrose), peptone and may be supplemented with an antibiotic that inhibits bacterial growth: chloramphenicol **(Pihet and Marot, 2013).**

Chromogenic media are media to which are added chromogenic substances that react with enzymes secreted by the yeasts, giving the colonies a particular coloration, variable according to the species (**Fig. 6**). Compared to the standard Sabouraud medium, the growth rate on chromogenic medium is slightly slower and the colonies are generally smaller in size. Examples of chromogenic media: Candida ID® 2, Candichrom®, ELITech Microbio, ChromID®, CHROMagar® Becton-Dickinson; OCCA®, Oxoid, CandiSelect®4 **(Pihet et Marot, 2013).**

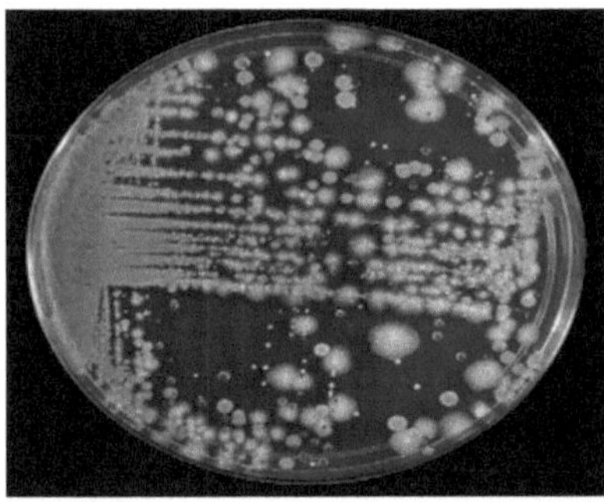

Figure 6. Association of different *Candida* species on the *Candida* ID®2 medium *(C. albicans and C. dubliniensis* in blue, *C. tropicalis,c lusitaniae, C. kefyr* in pink, C. *parapsilosis, C. glabrata* , etc. in white) **(Pihet and Marot, 2013).**

3.4. Yeast identification :

- **Blastosis (filamentous or germination) test:** is based on the fact that *C.albicans* (and also *C.dubiliensis*) produces in 3 hours at 37°C in human or animal serum, a germ tube from blastopores (**Fig.7**). This thin and flexuous germ tube does not represent any constriction at its base (unlike yeast pseudomycelium which is formed by budding, and represents a partition at the emergence of the daughter cell). This test therefore allows us to distinguish between ***C.albicans/C.dubliniensis*** and other *Candida* species **(Pihet and Marot, 2013).**

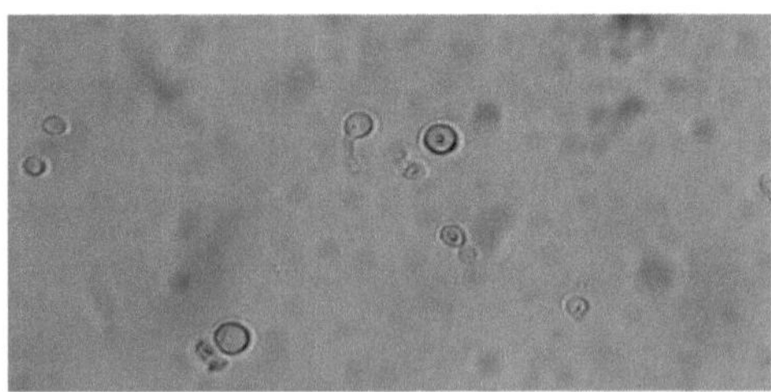

Figure 7. Germ tube of *Candida albicans in the* blastèse test (Photo taken at the HMPIT Laboratory)

□ **Chlamydosporulation test:** It is carried out by transplanting the strain in poor environments. Among these media we quote: Potato-Carrot, Potato-Carrot-Bile (PCB), Cornmeal Agar, Rize-Agar-Tween (RAT) and Agar-Tween (AT). Two techniques are described **(Pihet and Marot, 2013)**:

- **Tinned:** The medium cast in a 5 cm diameter petri dish is seeded in its center with a drop of yeast suspension and then covered with a slat. The dish is then incubated in an oven at 25-27°C. This technique can be used with all three types of media (RAT, AT and PCB).
- **In slide culture:** This technique is easier to perform on PCB medium. It consists in pouring on a slide, using a pipette, about 0.8 ml of PCB medium previously melted in a water bath, then inoculate the yeasts by making 2 streaks in the agar. Cover with a slide. Place the slide in a hermetically sealed box to avoid dissection. Incubate at 25-27°C for 24 hours.

□ **Biochemical tests**: These tests are based on the use of galleries, the principle of which consists of studying the assimilation of carbohydrates (auxanogram) and their fermentation (zymogram). Several commercialized galleries are widely used today in the identification of yeasts of which the most well known are: Auxacolor®, ID32C®, Fungifast®, Fongichrom® **(Pihet et Marot,2013).**

□ **Immunological tests:** The Bichrolatex® device is based on the principle of co-agglutination on slide. The reagent is a set of red colored latex particles sensitized by a monoclonal antibody recognizing a parietal antigen of *C. albicans.* The appearance of red agglutinates after a few minutes identifies *C. albicans* or *C. dubliniensis,* (**Fig. 8**). The differentiation between these two species is then based on a second device, the Bichrodubli® **(Pihet & Marot, 2013).**

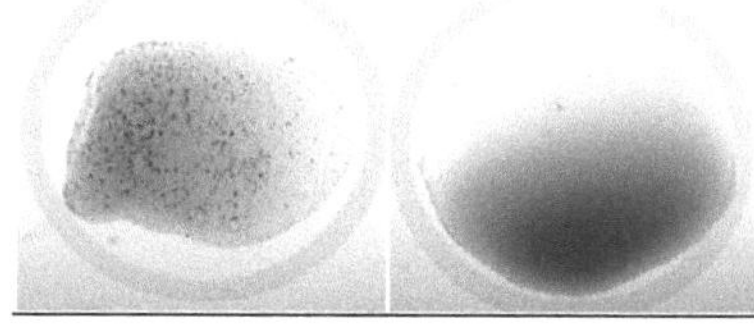

AB

Figure 8. Reaction of Bichrolatex *Albicans®* Fumouze_Source. A : Presence of *Candida albicans* B :Absence of *Candida albicans* **(Benkirane, 2014).**

□ **MALDI-TOF mass spectrometry: MALDI-TOF** mass spectrometry is considered today by microbiology committees to be the fastest, simplest, most reproducible and reliable technique for fungal identification. Genetic spectra of yeast proteins from cultured colonies are analyzed by comparison with reference spectra from databases. This technique is based on the separation of molecules transformed into ions, according to the m/z ratio (m=mass, z=charge) **(Bougnoux et *al.,* 2013).** Species identification by mass spectrometry is a three-phase process:

- A phase of ionization and desorption of the sample.
- A "flight" phase: allows to individualize the molecules of the sample according to their mass/charge ratio.
- A detection phase: a detector will transform the electrical information (produced by the ions at the end of their flight) into an electric current.

3.5. Antifungigram :

Its purpose is to determine in vitro the sensitivity of isolated strains to different families of antifungal agents. It allows the definition of a minimum inhibitory concentration (MIC) **(Pihet and Marot, 2013).**

Indeed, two expert committees, the CLSI "Clinical and laboratory standards institute" or more recently the NCCLS (National committee for clinical laboratory standards) for the United States and the EUCAST "European committee on antibiotic susceptibility testing" for Europe, propose standardized methods that serve as a reference for other tests. These techniques are based on the principle of microdilution in liquid medium. However, the use of these techniques remains limited to specialized laboratories. For this purpose, other in vitro sensitivity determination techniques have been developed, such as agar diffusion techniques (E-test and disc diffusion), microdilution techniques (Sensititre yeastOne, Vitek 2 AST-YS01) **(Table 2) (Abbes et *al.* , 2012) (Pihet and Marot, 2013).**

Table 2. Comparison of available sensitivity methods (**Abbes et** ***al.,*** **2012**).

Methods	Principle	Reading	Benefits	Disadvantages
CLSI	Microdilution or macrodilution in liquid medium	Visual	Reference Methods	Not marketed and Heavy
EUCAST	Microdilution in liquid media	Spectrophotometry		
E-TEST	Agar diffusion	Inhibitor ellipse	Standardized and Marketed	Expensive Difficult interpretation sometimes
Disc distributio n	Agar diffusion	Diameter of inhibition zone		Diffuculty of measurement CMI
Sensititre Yeast one	Microdilution in liquid media	Staining		Kit
Vitek 2 AST- YS01	Microdilution in liquid media	Spectrophotometry		Does not include echinocandins and the posaconazole

Materials and Methods

1. Hardware

1.1. Type, duration, location and population of study

This is a retrospective study that included 1058 vaginal swabs collected during three months between October and December 2018 in the laboratory of Parasitology-Mycology of the main military hospital of instruction in Tunis.

1.2. Criteria for inclusion

Our population is made up of women with symptoms suggestive of VSC or pregnant women undergoing a systematic check-up.

1.3. Criteria for non-inclusion

Sampling cannot be performed in any patient with at least one of these conditions:

- Patient during menstruation.
- Undergoing general or local anti-infectious treatment within the previous 14 days.
- Intimate toilet on the day of sampling or the day before.
- Sexual intercourse on the day of collection or within the last 72 hours.

1.4. Data Collection

For each patient, we collected clinical data from a questionnaire and biological data from the SYSLAB laboratory computer software.

In fact, the sampling room begins with an interrogation specifying: age, gestational age, parity, date of last menstrual period, history, presence or absence of clinical signs (leukorrhea, pruritus, dyspareunia) or urinary signs (**Appendix.1**). These clinical and mycological data are then entered into Excel and SPSS 22.0.

2. Methods

Mycological examination is essential to distinguish between colonization of the vaginal mucosa and an infection for which there are different treatments **(El Euch et *al.* ,2014).**

2.1. Sampling

Samples are taken by swabbing the lower third of the vagina and the vulval area in young girls. This swab is done with speculum in non-pregnant women to take samples of the endocervix and ectocervix for the bacteriology laboratory. These sterile swabs must be quickly examined and inoculated, not only to avoid alteration of the fungal elements, but also to detect possible vegetative forms of *Trichomonas vaginalis.*

2.2. Direct examination

Allows to give a first result immediately and to confirm the diagnosis of candidiasis by the detection of yeasts or pseudofilaments.

- Add 500 µl of physiological water to the swab.
- Shake the swab well, then place a few drops of this suspension between slide and sterile microscopic slide.
- Observe with an optical microscope at the objective (×40)

On direct examination, blastospores are observed which appear in a rounded or oval form, from 6 to 8 µ, in their longest length, budding or not, sometimes accompanied by pseudofilaments (**Fig.9**).

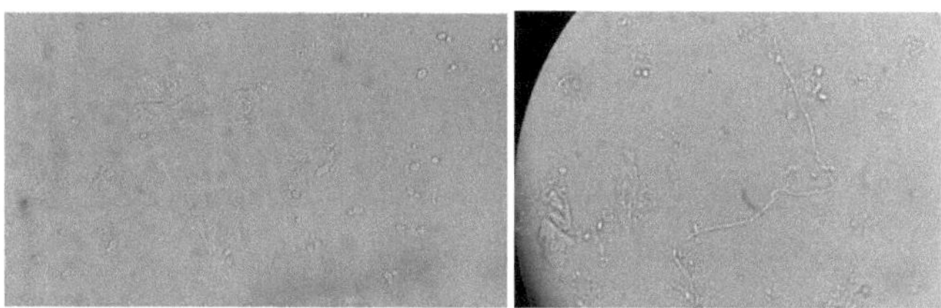

Figure 9. Blastospores (left) Pseudofilament (right)
(photos taken at the HMPIT laboratory)

2.3. Culture

Culture is the most sensitive method for the detection of *Candida* yeasts. It is performed on solid media.

□ **Isolation environments :**

S: Isolation is done on Sabouraud agar suitable for practically all fungi responsible for mycosis.

SC: Sabouraud medium added with antibiotic (chloramphenicol and gentamicin).

SCA : it is the SC medium with added actidione which is an antifungal agent that inhibits the development of saprophytic moulds and allows the differentiation of certain virulent yeast species (such as *C. albicans* which grows in the presence of actidione unlike *C. tropicalis*).

The composition and method of operation of these media are described in Appendix 2.

□ **Seeding technique**

The seeding is done according to the method of the dials: 1st dial is seeded using the completely discharged swab. The other dials are seeded with the sterilized buttoned Pasteur pipette.

□ **Incubation**

In an oven at 37°C for 48 hours. After incubation, the colonies are counted to estimate the abundance of fungal growth in numbers of + :

<10 colonies : +

10-50 colonies: ++

>50 well isolated

colonies : +++ Sheet

colonies : ++++

2.4. Identification

□ Macroscopic examination of the colonies: Observe the diameter, color and appearance of the colonies (**Fig.10**).

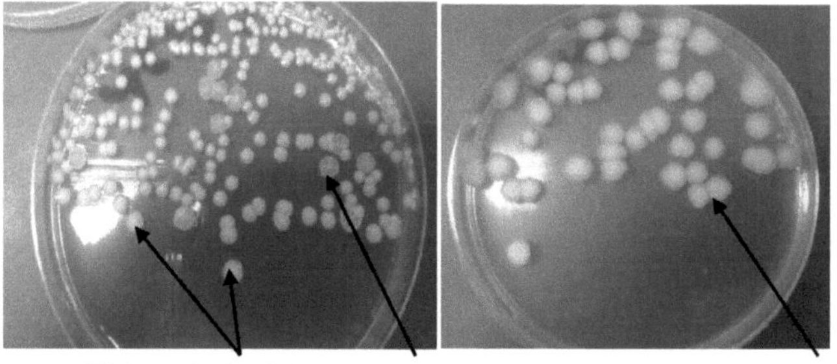

White coloniesColony dry pleatedColony dry beige

Figure 10. Different aspects of colonies after 48 h on SC medium (photos taken in the laboratory)

❖ **Identification process** (+ positive culture / - negative culture) :

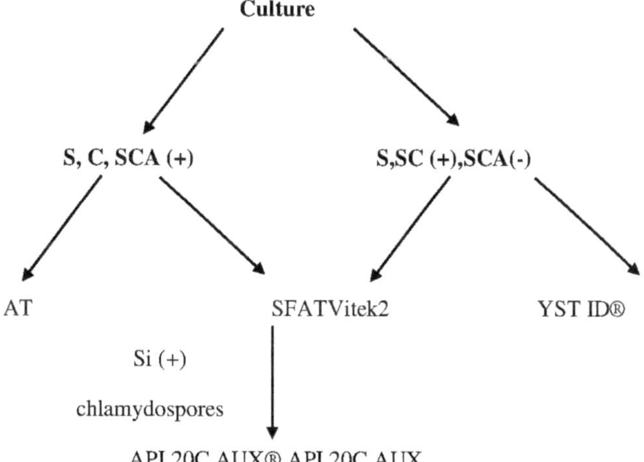

□ <u>Morphological criteria :</u>

❖ **Chlamydosporulation test**: This test consists of anaerobic **inoculation of the** yeasts on poor media such as Agar Tween (AT).

Colonies appearing on Sabouraud media will be transplanted in three striations on (AT), then covered with a slide. Incubation is done at 27°C in the oven for 24 hours.

The presence of terminal chlamydospores, which are thick-walled, globular spores measuring about 10 to 15 µm, is characteristic of the species *C.albicans* or *C.dubliniensis*. For other species, pseudofilaments or yeasts are observed. These three forms are illustrated in **Figure 11**.

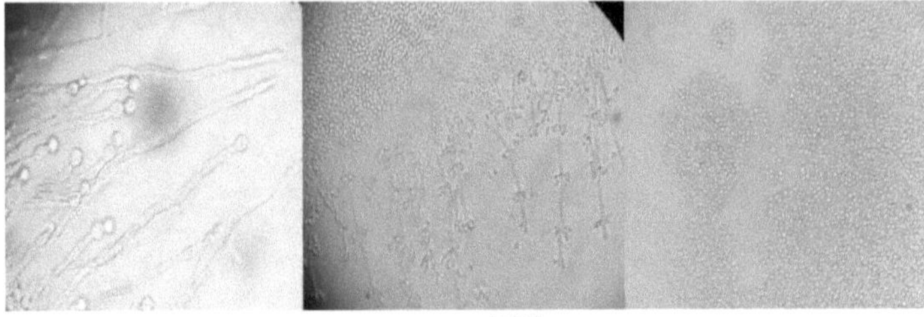

ABC

Figure 11. Observations of chlamydodspores A, pseudofilaments B , yeasts C , on AT medium (X40) (Pictures taken in the laboratory)

- **Transplanting on Sun Flower medium (SF)**

This medium is used to differentiate between *C. albicans* and *C. dubliniensis*. After incubation for 24 to 48 hours at 27°C, the colonies appear dry for *C. dubliniensis* and smooth for C. *albicans*. Microscopic examination of the colonies in a drop of physiological saline between slide and slide: Only C.*dubliniensis* has the capacity of chlamydosporulation on this medium.

The presence of chlamydospores requires the application of a second API 20C AUX® test to confirm the diagnosis of this species.

The composition and method of operation of these media are described in Appendix 3.

□ Biochemical criteria :

- **API 20C AUX® API 20C AUX**

This gallery consists of 20 wells (**Fig.12**) containing dehydrated substrates that allow 19 assimilation tests to be performed. The wells are inoculated with a minimum semi-agar medium and the yeasts grow only if they are able to use the corresponding substrate. These reactions are read by comparison with growth controls and identification is obtained using the Analytical Catalogue or identification software.

After 48 hours of incubation, or 72 hours (if the tests, especially glucose, are not clear after 48 hours), observe yeast growth compared to well 0, the negative control. A cup that is cloudier than the control indicates a positive reaction.

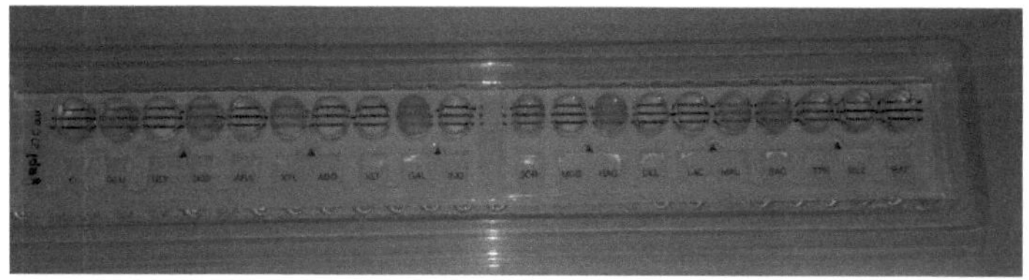

Figure 12. Api 20C Aux (Photo taken at the laboratory)

- **Auxanogram (Vitek2 YST ID®)**

The YST map is based on conventional biochemical methods and new substrates. There are 46 biochemical tests measuring carbon source utilization, nitrogen sources and enzyme activities. This growth is visualized by the turn of a pH indicator. The coloration thus changes from blue to yellow for sugars. For enzymes, a positive test results in a yellow coloration, a negative test remains colourless. The composition of the wells of the YST card is described in **Appendix 4**.

- Aseptically transfer 3.0 mL sterile saline solution (0.45 to 0.50% NaCl, PH 4.5 to 7) into a test tube (polystyrene)
- Transfer a sufficient number of morphologically similar colonies with the pasteur pipette into the tube of prepared saline solution. Adjust the yeast suspension between 1.8 and 2.2 Mc Farland using a DensiCHEKTM.
- Place the suspension tube and the YST card in the cassette (**Fig.13**).
- Insert the filled cassette into the Vitek 2 PLC (**Fig. 14**) and start the test.
- Results are obtained in about 18 hours.

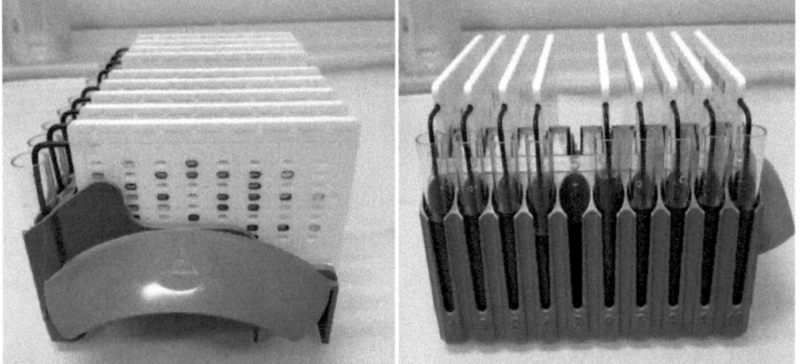

Figure 13. Vitek2 cassette filled with yeast suspensions and YST ID cards (photo taken in the laboratory).

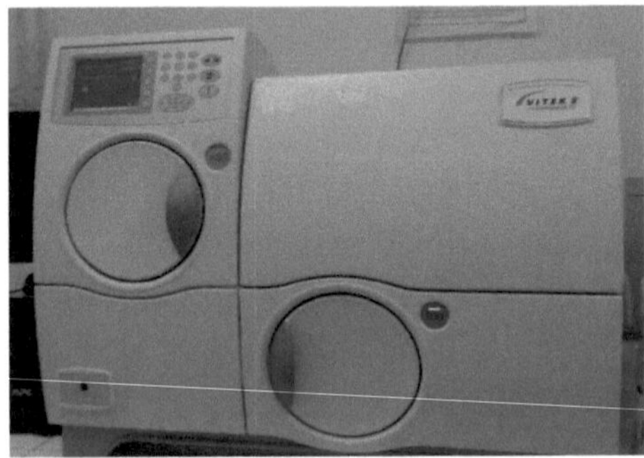

Figure 14. Vitek2® appliance

2.5. Antifungicide

We have limited ourselves to the study of two strains of *Candida, Candida albicans and Candida glabrata* since the antifungus test is not applicable to the mycology laboratory at HMPIT for vaginal swabs unless requested by the attending physician. The sensitivity of *Candida albicans* is tested by Vitek2 AST and of *Candida glabrata.*

by Vitek AST and E-test for Fluconazole.

- **Vitek ®2 AST**

Vitek 2 AST determines the MIC by the microdilution method (in µg/mL) in order to identify an interpretation criterion (Sensitive, Intermediate or Resistant) to facilitate the choice of therapy. Using the AST08 card, this system tests the *in vitro* sensitivity of *Candida* yeasts to **amphotericin B**, **fluconazole**, **fluorocytosine** and **voriconazole**, **Caspofungin**, **micafungin**.

Each card has a control well containing only microbiological culture medium. The other microwells contain preset concentrations of these antifungal agents and culture medium (**Appendix.5**).

This test consists of :

- Aseptically transfer 3 ml of sterile aqueous saline solution (0.45 to 0.5% Nacl, pH 4.5 to 7) into a transparent plastic (polystyrene) test tube.
- Using a pasteur pipette, transfer a sufficient number of identical colonies into the prepared saline tube. Adjust the yeast suspension between 1.8 and 2.2 Mc

Farland using a DensiCHEKTM.

- Transfer 280 µl of the prepared suspension into a second tube containing 3 ml of saline solution using a propette.
- Place the tube with the AST antibiotic susceptibility test card on the cassette and insert the assembly into the vitek®2 automated system (Fig. 27) to start the test.

• **E-test**

This method is based on the principle of diffusion in an agar medium. In practice, the E-test® strip of fluconazole, impregnated with an antifungal gradient, is applied to the surface of a medium previously inoculated with the strain to be tested, then the whole is incubated for 24 hours at 37°C. The MIC reading is taken at the intersection between the strip and the ellipsis of the fungal growth inhibition ellipsis.

Results

1. Prevalence of CVV

Out of a total of 1058 samples received, 273 showed a positive *Candida* yeast culture, for an overall prevalence of 25.8%.

2. Age distribution of the study population

The mean age of women with positive culture is 32 years (± 6.91) with extremes ranging from 20 to 64 years. The most affected age group is between 30 and 39 (**Fig.15**).

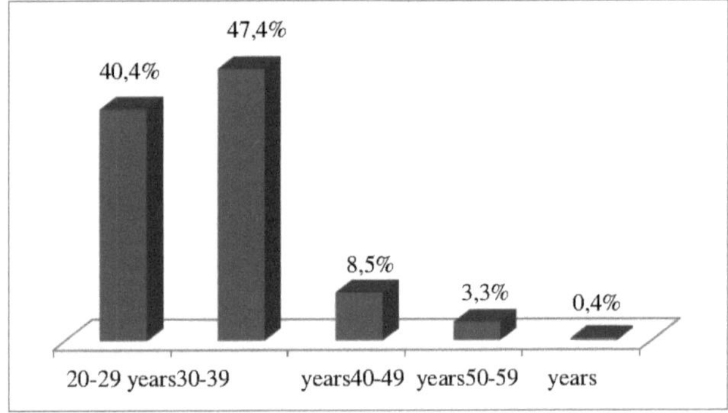

Figure 15. Distribution of patients with CVV by age group.

3. Distribution of the study population by pregnancy

In 67% of cases, patients with CVV were pregnant, the majority (46.3%) of whom were in the first trimester (**Figs.16 and 17**).

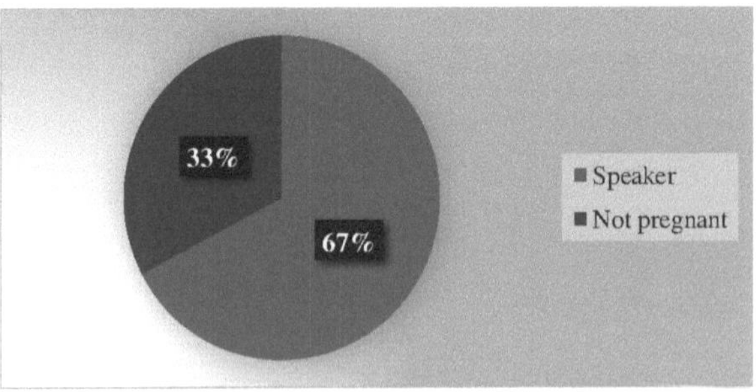

Figure 16. Distribution of CVV patients by pregnancy.

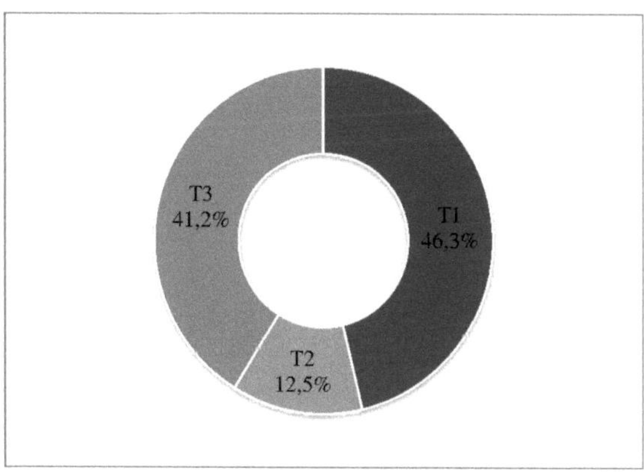

Figure 17. Prevalence of CVV by gestational age.

4. Patient Distribution by Clinical Signs

In 64.8% of cases, our patients had clinical manifestations dominated by leukorrhea followed by vulval pruritus and urinary burns (**Table 3**). They were asymptomatic in 96 cases (35.2%).

Table 3. Main clinical signs of patients with CVV.

Clinical events	Number of patients	Percentage (%)
Leucorrhea	157	57,6%
Vulvar pruritus	110	40,2%
Micturition burns	46	16,8%

5. Direct Examination Results

Direct examination is considered positive if it shows the presence of yeasts and/or pseudofilaments. Out of 1058 patients, 187 (17.7%) present a positive direct examination.

The sensitivity of this test is 68.5% (**Table 4**).

Table 4. Results of Direct Examination of Positive Samples

Direct examination		Number of patients	Percentage (%)
Positive	Yeast	110	40 ,3
	Pseudofilament	77	28,2
Negative		86	31,5
Total		**273**	100

6. Culture results

A quarter of the vaginal swabs collected during the study period had isolated ***Candida*** yeasts in culture (**Table 5**). Culture was abundant 3 + and 4 + in 191 samples, or 70% of cases (**Fig. 18**).

Table 5. Crop results for all samples

Culture	Number of patients	Percentage (%)
Positive	273	25 ,8
Negative	785	74,2
Total	1058	100

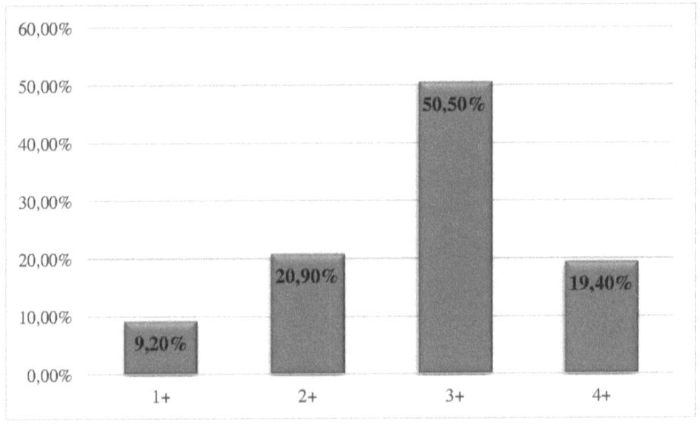

Figure 18. Distribution by Crop Abundance

7. Distribution of yeast genus *Candida* isolated in culture

The most isolated species in culture was *C. albicans in* 190 samples (66%) followed by *C. glabrata* in 77 samples (27%). **Figure 19** shows the different species isolated.

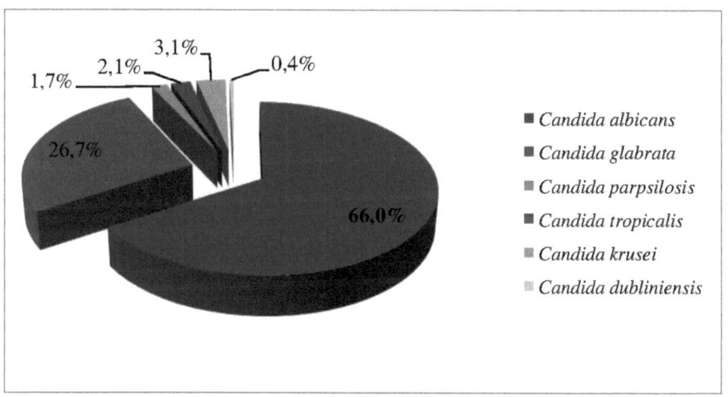

Figure 19. Main yeast species involved in VSC

8. Yeast associations in culture

In 18 cases (6.6%), ***Candida*** yeasts were in association with each other (14 cases) and with other yeasts: ***Trichosporon*** *(*1 case) and ***Saccharomyces*** *(*1 case) (**Fig.20**).

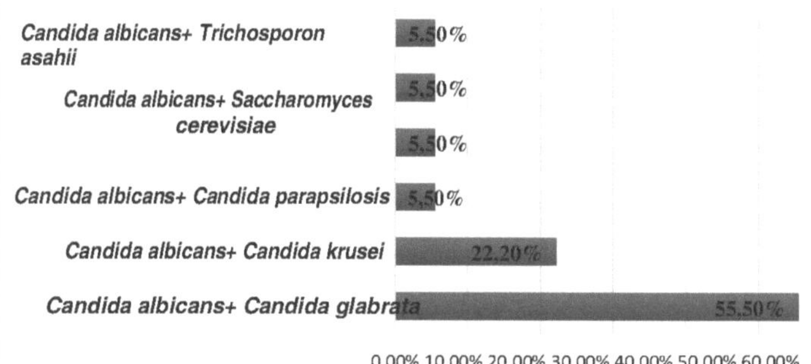

Figure 20: Frequencies of associations of isolated yeasts in culture.

9. Study of sensitivity to antifungal agents

- Study of the susceptibility of *Candida albicans* by Vitek®2 AST :

This strain is sensitive to fluconazole, voriconazole, flucytosine, caspofungin, micafungin and amphotericin B.

- Study of the susceptibility of *Candida glabrata* :

It is sensitive to voriconazole, flucytosine, caspofungin, micafungin and amphotericin B by Vitek®2 AST

The study of fluconazole sensitivity by the E-Test method, showed that *C. glabrata* is intermediateC~~MI~~ → 2 µg/mL (referring to EUCAST 2018 recommendations) (**Fig.21**).

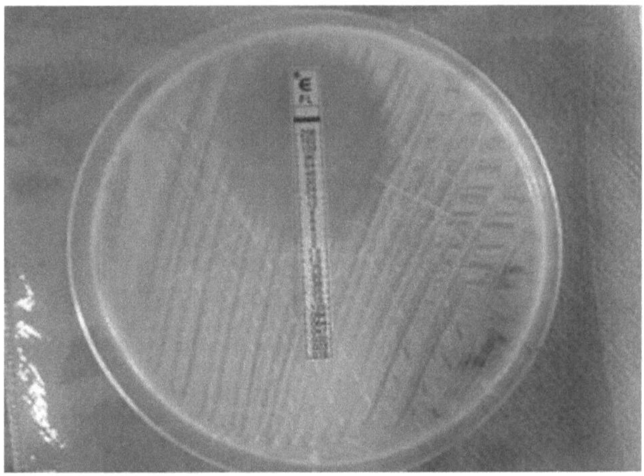

Figure 21. E-test: Sensitivity of *C. glabrata* to fluconazole (Photo taken at the HMPIT laboratory)

Discussion

VVC is a common gynecological infection of the reproductive tract affecting millions of women and is a global health problem **(Anane et *al.*, 2010) (Kechia et *al.*, 2015).**

According to studies carried out in different countries, the frequency of VSC varies from 6.5% to 38.9% (**Table 6**). The prevalence of VVC in our study is 25.8%. This is comparable to those reported by **Benchellal et *al* (2011)** (26%), **Hedayati et *al* (2014)** (28.2%), **Boughanmi (2015)** (31.81%). However a higher prevalence was

reported by **Anane et *al* (2010)** (36.39%) and **Ogouyèmi-Hounto et *al* (2014)** (38.9%). This difference can be explained by the variable number of vaginal samples taken by these different authors, the characteristics of the target population and the diagnostic methods used in each study.

Table 6. Prevalence of Vaginal Candidiasis Reported by Different Authors

Authors, year and location of study	Prevalence of CVVs
Our study	25,8%
Anane et *al*, 2010 Tunisia	36,39%
Dai et *al*, 2010 China	6,5%
Benchellal et *al*, 2011 Morocco	26%
Hedayati et *al*, 2014 Iran	28,2%
Ogouyèmi-Hounto et *al*, 2014 Benin	38,9%
Kechia et al, 2015 Yaoundé	35,52%
Boughanmi, 2015 Tunisia	31,81%
Mtibaa et *al*, 2017 Tunisia	32,87%

The incidence of VSC is low before puberty, but it is high in women of childbearing age and decreases after menopause, except in women using hormone replacement therapy **(Anane et *al.*, 2010) (Benchellal et *al.*, 2011) (Mtibaa et *al.*, 2017).** This was affirmed in our study where the most affected age group was between 30 and 39 years of age (47.4%), which is consistent with several studies

(**Table.7**). Indeed, this group is characterized by high sexual activity and estrogen load **(Ogouyèmi-Hounto et *al.*, 2014) (Kechia et *al.*, 2015).**

During pregnancy, the frequency of VSC increases from 26% to 67% (**Table.7**). According to our study, pregnant women represent 67% of the affected population with a gestational age distribution of 46.3% and 41.2% in Q1 and Q3 respectively. However, the study by **Benchellal et *al* (2011)** reported frequencies of 8%,38%,35% for Q1, Q2 and Q3 respectively. Similarly, the study by **Kechia et *al* (2015)** found a prevalence of 36.22% in Q2 and 52.63% in Q3.

Indeed, this period is characterized by a hormonal imbalance leading to a drop in vaginal pH, which favors the implantation of *Candida* yeasts. In addition, the increase in estrogen levels during pregnancy or the procreation period leads to the multiplication of *Candida yeasts* and their adhesion to epithelial cells **(Amouri et *al.*, 2010) (Ogouyèmi-Hounto et *al.*, 2014).**

Table 7. Mean Age and Pregnancy in CVV Studies

Authors, year of study	**Average age (years)**	**Percentage of Pregnancy (%)**
Noted study	32	67,3
Anane et *al*, 2010	32,47	53,1
Benchellal et *al*, 2011	29	26
Ogouyèmi-Hounto et *al*, 2014	29,83	51,5
Boughanmi, 2015	31,19	33,82
Mtibaa et *al*, 2017	33	44,1

Pruritus, vulvar burns and dyspareunia are the major symptoms of VSC. Sometimes they are associated with leucorrhoea of curdled appearance, thick adhesions to the vaginal mucosa of variable abundance. Dysuria, erythema, edema of the vulva, fissures or excoriations may also be observed **(Benchellal et *al.*, 2011). The** onset of pruritus (itching) can be explained by the invasion of epithelial cells of the genital tract by *Candida* yeasts. Inflammation is the result of the action of a toxin or enzyme involved in the pathogenesis of *Candida* infection **(Hedayati et *al.*, 2014).** In our series, leucorrhoea is the most frequent sign (57.6%) followed by vulvar pruritus (40.2%) and urinary burns (16.8%). Leukorrhea and vulvar pruritus are the most common clinical signs described in the studies. However, urinary burns are poorly reported in the literature with a variable percentage from one study to another. The symptoms reported by different authors are summarized in **Table 8**.

Table 8. Clinical symptoms during VSC reported by different authors

	Leucorrhea (%)	**Vulvar pruritus** (%)	**Urinary burns** (%)	**Dyspareunia** (%)
Our study	57,6	40,2	19,9	-
Anane et *al*, 2010	89,70	77,28	-	49 ,12
Benchellal et *al*, 2011	69,2	65,4	27	50
Ogouyèmi-Hounto et *al*, 2014	51,9	51,9	-	36,5
Kechia et *al*, 2015	60,28	61,70	-	-
Boughanmi, 2015	63,28	48,96	27,49	-
Mtibaa et *al*, 2017	72,25	63,25	24,92	32,25

(-): Not reported in the study.

In our study, 35.2% of women with CVV were asymptomatic. Indeed, *Candida* yeasts can be isolated from 20% of the genital tract of asymptomatic, healthy women of childbearing age **(Rodríguez-Cerdeira et *al.*, 2018).**

In addition to the clinical signs suggestive of CVV, the diagnosis must be confirmed by mycological examination **(Mtibaa et *al.*, 2017).** The latter includes a direct examination and culture, the positivity frequencies of which are 17.7% and 25.8% respectively in our study. The direct examination has a sensitivity that varies from 67% to 92% depending on the literature, illustrated in **Table 9.**

This difference may be caused by poor swabbing technique or false negatives in the microscopic reading of the direct examination.

Table 9. Sensitivity of SA reported in the literature

	ED sensitivity (%)
Our study	68 ,5
Anane et *al,* 2010	67,67
Hedayati et *al,* 2014	86,36
Ogouyèmi-Hounto et *al,* 2014	92,15
Mtibaa et *al,* 2017	73,23

Indeed, the culture allows the recovery of "false negatives" from the direct examination. However, culture remains the most sensitive and accurate method of diagnosis and also allows species identification based on macroscopic criteria **(Anane et *al.,* 2010) (Hedayati et *al.,* 2014).** Of the 25.8% that had a positive culture, almost 70% had an abundant culture of more than +++, which provides information on infection. The majority of CVVs are caused by *Candida albicans.* In our study, *Candida albicans* was isolated in 66% of cases followed by *Candida glabrata* in 26.7%. This is consistent with the results of all the studies presented in **Table 10,** which reports a prevalence of *Candida albicans* ranging from 42% to 86%. The predominance of this species is explained by its ability to adhere to the vaginal mucosa due to the presence of vaginal cellular receptors of the *Candida* ligand, which allows the expression of virulence factors.

Recently, there has been an increase in *non-albican* species according to the literature (**Table.10**). Among these, *Candida glabrata* has been the most commonly associated with CVV with an isolation rate of 8% to 26% depending on the studies. This increased prevalence of *non-albicans candida* is due to incomplete local or systemic treatment regimens, self-prescribed antifungal agents and prolonged use of antifungal agents to prevent recurrence of CVV **(Hedayati et *al.,* 2014).**

Candida dubliniensis is present in 0.4% of our isolates. This rate is significantly lower than that reported by **Hedayati el *al* (2014):** 16.4%. This rare species, previously described as being specific to HIV+ subjects and especially in the oral cavity, is present in the vagina of immunocompetent patients.

Table 10. Prevalence of different *Candida* species reported in Literature

	Our study	**Anane et *al*, 2010**	**Hedayati et *al*, 2014**	**Kechia et *al*, 2015**	**Boughanmi , 2015**	**Mtibaa et *al*, 2017**
Candida albicans	66%	81,16%	42,5%	86,52%	73,57%	76,61%
Candida glabrata	26,7%	12,62%	21,9%	8,51%	19,27%	17,18%
Candida parapsilosis	1,7%	1,17%	-	-	0,83%	-
Candida tropicalis	2,1%	1,55%	-	3,55%	0,72%	1,4%
Candida krusei	3,1%	1,36%	-	0,71%	0,72%	1,54%
Candida kefyr	-	1,36%	8,2%	0,71%	0,1%	0,56%
Candida dubliniensis	0,4%	-	16,4%	-	-	-
candida guilliermondii	-	0,39%	2,7%	-	-	-
Candida pintolopesii	-	-	8,2%	-	-	-

(-): Not reported in the study.

In our study, cultures showed in 18 cases an association of two yeast species. In 55.5% of the cases, it was an association of *Candida albicans* and *Candida glabrata.* **Hedayati et *al* (2014)** reported the association of *Candida yeast* genus in the cultures of CVV patients in seven cases out of 234, 71% of which was an association between *C.albicans* and *C.glabrata.*

Some *non-albican* species such as *C. glabrata* respond poorly to azole agents, notably fluconazole **(Abbess et *al.*,2015).** In our study, a strain of *Candida glabrata* has an intermediate sensitivity to fluconazole. In the US study by **Sobel et *al* (2003) of** 44 isolates of *Candida glabrata*, 4.5% were resistant and only 9.1% of the strains were susceptible to fluconazole.

Conclusion and Outlook

Conclusion

CVV is a common gynecological infection of the reproductive tract that affects millions of women each year. It manifests itself through clinical signs that interfere with a woman's normal life.

This study demonstrates the relatively important place of vulvovaginal candidiasis in gynecological infections.

In fact, CVV affects 25.8% of patients referred to the parasitology-mycology service at the main military training hospital in Tunis. The major pathogens responsible for this pathology are *Candida albicans* and *Candida glabrata* in 66% and 26.7% of cases respectively.

The management of CVV requires a precise diagnosis based on a good interrogation, clinical and mycological examination. The latter makes it possible to differentiate between colonization and vaginal candidiasis infection, among other things the precise identification of the species in question, which could make it possible to avoid the antifungal agent for which innate resistance is known.

Perspectives

At present, an emergence of *non-albicans* species can be noted following the abuse of azole treatments. These species, in particular *Candida glabrata* and *Candida krusei,* are more resistant to antifungal agents.

For a better management of this pathology it is necessary to :

- Take a mycological sample with direct examination and culture (specifying the number of colonies and the species involved).
- Look for all known predisposing factors and treat them.

Eventually, a better understanding of host defense factors specific to the vagina will help in understanding susceptibility to opportunistic infections.

Bibliographical references

Abbes, S.A., Trabelsi, H.O., Amouri, I.M., Sallemi, H.A., Nej, S.O., Chikhrouhou, F.A., Makni, F.A., Ayadi, A.L. (2012). Methods for the study of in vitro sensitivity of *Candida spp.* to antifungal agents. *Annals of Clinical Biology* 70 (6): 635-642.

Amouri, I., Abbes, S., Sellami, H., Makni, F., Sellami, A., Ayadi, A. (2010). La candidose vulvo-vaginale revue. *Journal of Medical Mycology* 20 (2): 108-115.

Anane, S., Kaouech, E., Zouari, B., Belhadj, S., Kallel, K., Chaker, E. (2010). Vulvovaginal candidiasis: risk factors and clinical and mycological particularities. *Journal of Medical Mycology* 20(1) :36-41.

Anofel (2017). Chapter 5 - Diagnosis by nature of the sample. In: *Medical Parasitology and Mycology - Guide des Analyses et des Pratiques Diagnostiques.* Eds Botterel,F.R., Dardé, M.L., Debourgogne, A., Delhaes, L., Houzé, S., Morio, F., Kauffmann-Lacroix, C., Roques, C. p :95-155.

Benchellal, M., Guelzim, K., Lemkhente, Z., Jamili, H., Dehainy, M., Rahali Moussaoui, D., El Mellouki, W., Sbai Idrissi, K., Lmimouni, B. (2011). Vulvo-vaginal candidiasis at the Mohammed V Military Training Hospital (Morocco). *Journal of Medical Mycology* 21(2): 106-112.

Benkirane, H. (2014). Evaluation of the bichrolatex Albicans® VERSUS filamentation test for the identification of *Candida* yeasts. Doctoral thesis in Pharmacy, Faculty of Medicine and Pharmacy of RABAT, 56 pages.

Boughanmi, M.(2015). Vaginal yeast and germ infections and their associations. Doctoral thesis in Pharmacy, Faculty of Pharmacy of Monastir, 61 pages.

Bougnoux, M.E., Angebault, C.E, Leto, J.U, Beretti, J.L. (2013). Identification of yeasts by MALDI-TOF mass spectrometry. *Revue Francophone Des Laboratoires 2013* (450): 63-69.

Cassone, A. (2014). Vulvovaginal *Candida albicans* infections: pathogenesis, immunity and vaccine prospects. *An International Journal of Obstetrics &*

Gynaecology 122 : 785-794.

D.Parent. (2017). Female genital mucosa. In: *Dermatology and Sexually Transmitted Infections (6th edition).* p: 905-915.

Dai, Q.I., Hu, L.I., Jiang, Y.O., Shi, H.U., Liu, J.I., Zhou, W.E., Shen, C.H., Yang, H.U. (2010). An epidemiological survey of bacterial vaginosis, vulvovaginal candidiasis and trichomoniasis in the Tibetan area of Sichuan Province, China. *European Journal of Obstetrics & Gynecology and Reproductive Biology 150* (2): 207-209.

De Chauvin, M. F. (2009). Vulvovaginal candidiasis. In: *Sexually Transmitted Infections.* p:134-139.

Defosse, T. A., Le Govic, Y., Courdavault, V., Clastre, M., Vandeputte, P., Chabasse, D., Bouchara, J.P., Giglioli-Guivarc'h, N., Papon, N. (2018). CTG clade (*Candida* clade) yeasts: biology, human health implications and biotechnology applications. *Journal of Medical Mycology* 28 (2): 257-268.

Develoux, M., Bretagne, S. (2005). Various candidiasis and yeast infections. *EMC - Infectious Diseases* 2 (3): 119-139.

EGGIMANN, P., PITTET, D. (2002). Candidates in resuscitation. *Resuscitation* 11(3) : 209–221.

El Euch, D.A. (2014). Superficial mycoses. *In: Infectious Dermatology.* Eds. Trojjet, S.O., Mokni, M.O., Feuilhade de Chauvin, M.A. p: 185-198.

Godha, K.E., Tucker, K. M., Biehl, C.O., Archer, D. F., Mirkin, S.E. (2017). Human vaginal pH and microbiota: an update. *Gynecological Endocrinology* 34 (6): 451- 455.

Greenbaum, S.H., Greenbaum, G.I., Moran-Gilad, J.A., Weintruab, A.Y. (2018). Ecological dynamics of the vaginal microbiome in relation to health and disease. *American Journal of Obstetrics and Gynecology 220 (4): 324-335.*

Hedayati, M. T., Taheri, Z.A., Galinimoghadam, T.A., Aghili, S. R., Yazdani Cherati, J., & Mosayebi, E.L. (2015). Isolation of Different Species of *Candida* in Patients With Vulvovaginal Candidiasis From Sari, Iran. *Jundishapur Journal of Microbiology* 8.

Holanda, A. R., Fernandes, C. S., Bezerra, C. M., Ferreira, Â. F., Holanda, R. R., Holanda, C. P., Milan, E. P. (2007). Vulvovaginal candidiasis: symptomatology, risk factors and concomitant anal colonization. *Revista Brasileira de Ginecologia e Obstetrícia,* 29(1) :3-9.

Kechia, F.A., Dohbit, J.S., Kouotou, E.A., Iwewe, S.Y., Dzoyem, J.P., Mbopuwouo, N.M., Monamele, C.G., Moyou , S.R. (2015). Epidemiological and etiological profile of vulvo-vaginal candidiasis in pregnant women in Yaoundé. *Health Sci Dis* 16: 1-6.

Masand, D. L., Patel, J.A., Gupta, S.W. (2015). Utility of Microbiological Profile of Symptomatic Vaginal Discharge in Rural Women of Reproductive Age Group. *Journal of clinical and diagnostic research* 9: 04-07.

Miller, E.A., Beasley, D.E., Dunn, R.R., Archie, E.A. (2016). Lactobacilli Dominance and Vaginal pH: Why Is the Human Vaginal Microbiome Unique?. *Frontiers in Microbiology: 1936.*

Mtibaa, L, Fakhfakh, N, Kallel, A, Belhadj, S, Belhaj Salah, N, Bada, N, Kallel, K (2017). Vulvovaginal candidiasis: etiology, symptomatology and risk factors. *J Mycol Med* 27 (2): 153-158.

Ogouyèmi-Hounto, A., Adisso, S., Djamal, J., Sanni, R., Amangbegnon, R., Biokou-Bankole, B., Kinde Gazard, D., Massougbodji, A. (2014). Place of vulvo-vaginal candidiasis during low-genital infections and associated risk factors in women in Benin. *Journal of Medical Mycology* 24: 100-105.

Palková, Z.D., Váchová, L.I. (2016). Yeast cell differentiation. *Lessons from pathogenic and non-pathogenic yeasts.* Seminars in Cell & Developmental Biology 57: 110-119.

Papon, N.I., Courdavault, V.I., Clastre, M.A., Bennett, R.J. (2013). Emerging and Emerged Pathogenic *Candida* Species: Beyond the Candida albicans Paradigm. *Journal.ppat* 9 (9).

Pihet, M.A., Marot, A.G. (2013). Biological diagnosis of candidiasis. *Revue Francophone Des Laboratoires* 2013 (450): 47-61.

Foal, D.A. (2013). *Candida albicans*, plasticity and pathogenesis. *Revue Francophone des Laboratoire* 2013 450: 37-46.

Rodríguez-Cerdeira, C.A., Gregorio, M.C., Molares-Vila, A.L., López-Barcenas, A.D., Fabbrocini, G.A., Bardhi, B.R., Sinani, A.R., Sánchez-Blanco, E.L., Arenas-Guzmán, R.O., Hernandez-Castro, R.I. (2018). Biofilms and vulvovaginal candidiasis. *Colloids and Surfaces B: Biointerfaces* 174: 110-125.

Seifi, Z.A., Zarei Mahmoudabadi, A.L., Zarrin, M.A. (2015). Extracellular Enzymes and Susceptibility to Fluconazole in *Candida* Strains Isolated From Patients With Vaginitis and Healthy Individuals. *Jundishapur Journal of Microbiology* 8 (3).

Sharma, J.E., Rosiana, S.I., Razzaq, I.Q, Shapiro, R.E. (2019). Linking Cellular Morphogenesis with Antifungal Treatment and Susceptibility in *Candida* Pathogens. *Journal of Fungi 5 (1).*

Sobel, J.D., Zervos, M., Reed, B.D., Hooton, T., Soper, D., Nyirjesy P., Heine, M.W., Willems, J., Panzer, H. (2003). Fluconazole susceptibility of vaginal isolates obtained from women with complicated *Candida* vaginitis: clinical implications *Antimicrobial Agents and Chemotherapy* 47: 34-38.

Tachedjian, G.I., Aldunate, M.U., Bradshaw, C. S., Cone, R.A. (2017). The role of lactic acid production by probiotic *Lactobacillus* species in vaginal health. *Research in Microbiology 168(9-10) :782-792.*

Tsui, C.H., Kong, E.F., Jabra-Rizk, M.A. (2016). Pathogenesis of *Candida* albicans biofilm. *Pathogens and Disease* 74 (4).

Van Schalkwyk, J.U., Yudin, M. H., Allen, V.I., Bouchard, C.E., Boucher, M.A., Boucoiran, I.S., Caddy, S.H., Castillo, E.L., Murphy, K.E., Ogilvie, G.I., Paquet, C.A.(2015). Vulvovaginitis: Screening and management of trichomoniasis, vulvovaginal candidiasis and bacterial vaginosis. *Journal of Obstetrics and Gynaecology Canada* 320: 587-596.

Appendices

Appendix 1. HMPIT Fact Sheet

Date: ………………

Name : ……….: ……………………:……………………………….. .

Profession : . ……………………………Address :……………………………………… .

Pregnancy: ... …………DDR: Number ....of pregnancies/children …………

Contraception :

OraleDIVOther

Underlying pathology: ………………………………………………………… . .

Therapeutics in progress: …………………………………………………………. . .

Clinic :

LeukorrheaPruritBulb urination

Leucorrhoees : Color

Fetishes

Abundant

Others :...

Appendix 2. Composition and method of preparation of the culture media used

Sabouraud(S) Environment

Sabouraud Agar... ....45g/L

Boil ....

Autoclaving for 15 min at 120°C ....

Allow to cool ....

Medium Sabouraud chloramphenicol Agar(C)

Sabouraud chloramphenicol Agar.. 45g/L

Boil... ...

Allow to cool and then add :

2 vials of gentamicin ....

2 vials of colimycin

Autoclave for 15 min at 120°C.. .

Allow to cool ....

Medium Sabouraud chloramphenicol Actidione (Agar) (A)

Sabouraud Chloramphenicol Actidione Agar ... 45g/L Boil it up

....

Allow to cool and then add:

2 phials of gentamicin... .

2 bottles colimycin ....

Autoclave for 15 min at 120°C.. .

Allow to cool...

The pH of ***these three media is equal to 6.5***

Appendix 3. Composition and method of preparation of media used for the identification of Candida yeasts.

Middle Agar Tween (AT)

Agar ... 18g/L

Boil...

Allow to cool ....

Add 10 ml of Tween 80, shake well. ....

Autoclaving for 15 min at 120°C ....

Allow to cool ....

Sunflower Medium (S.F)

Sunflower powder50g/L

Boil for 30 min. ....

Filter then add: Agar... .... 16g/L

Glucose 30%35 ....5ml

Autoclaving for 15 min at 120°C ....

Allow to cool..

Appendix 4. Composition of the wells of the VITEK® 2 YST ID® card

Well	Test	Mnemonic	Dosage / Wells
3	L-Lysine ARYLAMIDASE	LysA	0.0228 mg
4	Assimilation of L-MALATE	IMLTa	0.15 mg
5	Leucine ARYLAMIDASE	Leu A	0.0234 mg
7	ARGININE	ARG	0.15 mg
10	Assimilation of ERHYTHRITOL	ERYa	0.3 mg
12	Assimilation of glycerol	GlyLa	0.16 µl
13	Tyrosine-Arylamidase	TyrA	0.0276 mg
14	Beta-N-Acetyl GLUCOSAMINIDASE	BNAG	0.0408 mg
15	Assimilation of ARBUTINE	ARBa	0.3 mg
18	Amygdalin Assimilation	AMYa	0.3 mg
19	Assimilation of D-Galactose	dGALa	0.3 mg
20	Assimilation of GENTABIOSIS	GENa	0.3 mg
21	Assimilation of D-GLUCOSE	dGLUa	0.3 mg
23	Assimilation of Lactose	LACa	0.96 mg
24	Assimilation of Methyl-AD-GLUCOPYRANOSIDE	MAdGa	0.3 mg
26	Assimilation of D-CELLOBIOSIS	dCELa	0.3 mg
27	Gama-GLUTAMYL-Transferase	GGT	0.0228 mg
28	Assimilation of D-MALTOSE	dMALa	0.3 mg
29	Assimilation of D-RAFFINOSIS	dRAFa	0.3 mg
30	PNP-N-Acetyl-BD-GALACTOSAMINIDASE1	NAGA1	0.0306 mg
32	Assimilation of D-Mannose	dMNEa	0.3 mg
33	Assimilation of D-MELIBIOSIS	dMELa	0.3 mg
34	Assimilation of D-MELIZITOSIS	dMLZa	0.3 mg
38	Assimilation of L-SORBOSE	ISBEa	0.3 mg
39	Assimilation of L-RHAMNOSIS	IRHAa	0.3 mg
40	Assimilation of XYLITOL	XLTa	0.3 mg
42	Assimilation of L-SORBITOL	dSORa	0.1875 mg
44	Assimilation of SUCROSE/SUCROSE	SACa	0.3 mg
45	UREASE	URE	0.15 mg
46	AlPHA-GLCOSIDASE	AGLU	0.036 mg
47	Assimilation of D-TURANOSIS	DTURa	0.3 mg
48	Assimilation of D-TREALOSIS	DTREa	0.3 mg
49	Assimilation of NITRATE	NO3a	0.03 mg
51	Assimilation of L-ARABINOSIS	IARAa	0.3 mg
52	Assimilation of D-GALACTURONATE	dGATa	0.15 mg
53	Hydrolysis of the ESCULINE	ESC	0.225 mg
54	Assimilation of L-GLUTAMATE	IGLTa	0.15 mg
55	Assimilation of D-XYLOSE	dXYLa	0.3 mg
56	Assimilation of DL-LACTATE	LATa	0.15 mg
58	Assimilation of ACETATE	ACEa	0.15 mg
59	Assimilation of CITRATE (SODIUM)	CITa	0.15 mg
60	Assimilation of GLUCURONATE	GRTas	0.15 mg
61	Assimilation of L-PROLINE	IPROa	0.15 mg
62	Assimilation of 2-CETO-GLUCONATE	2KGa	0.15 mg
63	Assimilation of NACETYL-GLUCOSAMINE	NAGa	0.15 mg
64	Assimilation of D-GLUCONATE	dGNTa	0.15 mg

Appendix 5. Composition of the VITEK® 2 AST card

Numerical values are expressed in µg/L.

Antibiotic	Code	Concentran §	Open range ≤	Open range ≥	Indications for use FDA
Amphoterice B	ab01n	1 ; 4 ; 16 ; 32	0,25	16	N/A
Caspofungine	case02n	0 ; 12 ; 0,5 ; 2 ; 8	0,125	8	*C.albicans, C.krusei C.parapsilosis C.tropicalis C.guillermandi C.glabrata*
Fluconazole	flu02n	2 ; 4 ; 8 ; 16 ; 32 ; 64	0,5	64	*C.dubliniensis C.albicans, C.parapsilosis C.tropicalis C.guillerma ndi C.lusitaniae*
Flucytosine	fct02n	1 ; 4 ; 16 ; 32	1	64	*C.albicans C.dublinien sis C.glabrata C.guillerma ndi C.lusitaniae , C.parapsilo sis C.tropicalis*
Micafungine	mcf02n	0,06 ; 0,25 ; 1 ; 4	0,06	8	N/A
VoriconazoleSDD	vrc02n	0,5 ; 1 ; 4 ; 8	0,12	8	*C.albicans, C.krusei C.parapsilosis C.tropicalis C.lusitaniae C.guillermandi*

§ : Concentration of equivalent standard method by efficiency.

**N/A: No FDA specific user indication available. FDA: US Food and Drug Administration.

SDD: Dose-dependent sensitivity (SDD) defined as intermediate(I).

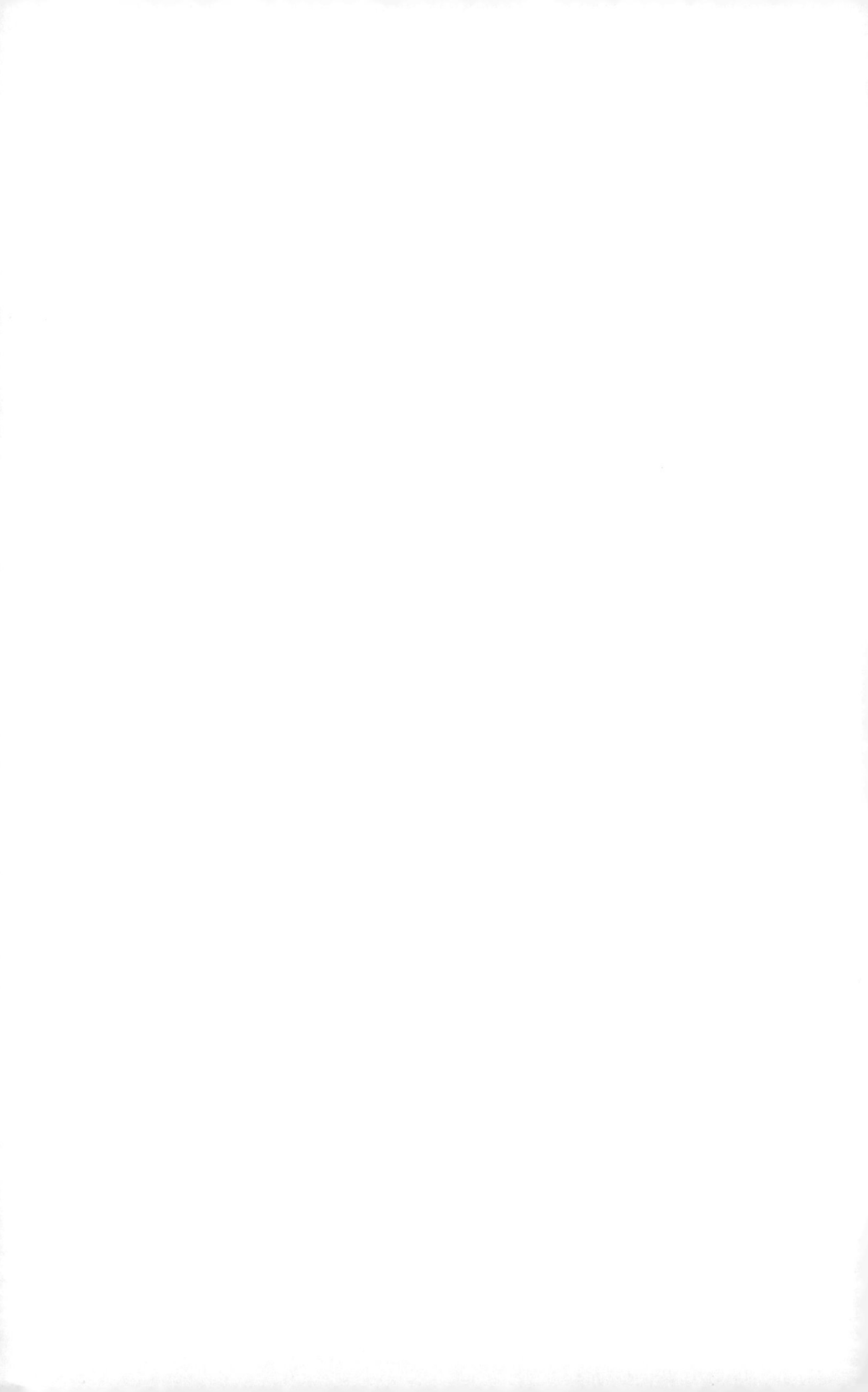

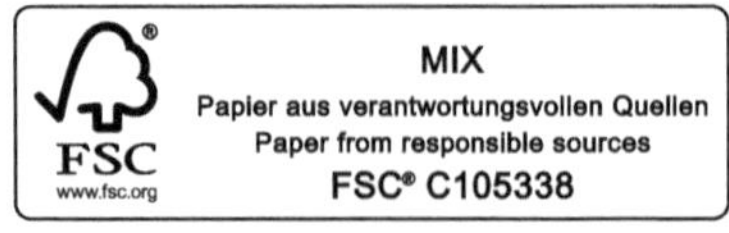

Printed by Books on Demand GmbH, Norderstedt / Germany